Inside Medicine

By Patrick D. Abiuso MD, FACP

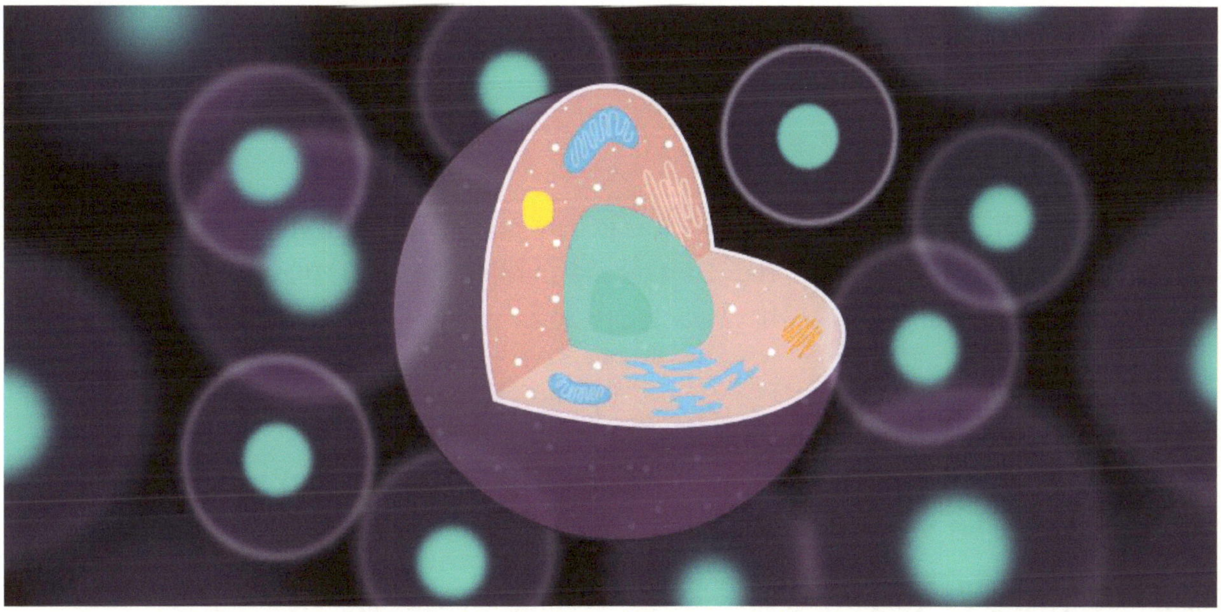

INTRODUCTION

I am a board certified Internal Medicine physician who has been actively involved in the medical community for 50 years. I've served many different roles during my career, but my primary focus has always been caring for my patients' health and well-being. Through thousands of patient encounters (many of these patients have been with me for decades) I have learned and grown to consider these people not only my patients, but also some of my friends and even family.

At the time of this writing, I continue to see patients full time. Planning retirement and wanting to impart some information to a larger audience prompted me to consolidate my thoughts into this book. Within these pages are concepts and conversations that I have found helpful for my patients through the decades.

This book is for the average person. My goal is to give information regarding how to stay healthy and help avoid some serious consequences of diseases. To do this, most patients have to navigate the health system to some degree. I will try to give you some understanding of the current system in the United States and how to negotiate it.

PREFACE

In one of my earliest memories as a child, I was in bed, not feeling well, and my mother called a physician to come to our house for me. He gave me an injection and I suddenly felt better. This man became my hero and I knew what I wanted to do as an adult. Medicine would become my profession.

Although we came from a modest family, and none of my family members had even attended college at that point, my mother continually reinforced to me that if I worked hard and put my mind to it, I could become anything I wanted.

With that in mind, I started to journey towards becoming a physician.

I did well in academics and sports through high school and college. I worked hard, keeping in mind at all times that my goal was to be able to get into medical school. I finally applied and was accepted. It was a lifelong dream come true. However, at the same time, the Vietnam draft occurred and there was a lottery system. I was worried that all the time and hard work to get into medical school would be in vain. I heard each number called and, finally, I realized that I was past the required number and would be able to proceed with my education.

This meant I ended up alone, for the first time in my life, in an inner city for my medical school training. Aside from the hardest academic workload I'd ever had, making the transition in the city and away from my family was difficult. My parents had worked multiple jobs to get us into the suburbs where I grew up most of my life. The inner city was quite a different place. Thank goodness for the new friends I made who were supportive. We all realized we needed to work together to get through.

There were a few funny situations, too. Once, we had this aggressive delivery driver, unsure where he was going, burst angrily into the room where we were doing an autopsy. He promptly passed out when he saw where he was and realized what we were doing! Other times, when we would leave the hospital we would have street vendors trying to sell used watches one day but fresh fish from the trunk of their cars the next!

Needless to say, it was a big adjustment and my classmates and I muddled through the four years together. And at the end of the time, my dream came true, and I was awarded a Doctor of Medicine degree. Then it was time to go out and practice the profession.

With this came internship and residency. During the first six months, there were times I would wake up with soaking sweats and anxiety, because I now realized that decisions I made would affect people's lives. Although I felt I had solid book knowledge, applying it to everyday patient life was challenging.

We had a tight schedule every third night and, in between, we tried to work in the emergency room to make some money to survive. I felt like I've seen some things I never should have seen or, rather, would have been better off without seeing. Things such as a coke bottle in a patient's rectum leave little to the imagination, but you truly haven't lived until you've looked into someone's ear and have seen a cockroach staring back at you!

These were the times when we learned to apply what we'd learned in the books to actual hands-on patient-care. Luckily, we had residents and mentors who were able to help us along the way until we were confident enough to make our own decisions for the patient.

Following that, we had our surgical rotation. Essentially, what would happen was all the good surgeries would go to the chief resident. Next best would go to the resident. The next down the line would go to the intern. And the students, we did all the scut work. So we found ourselves debriding patients, suturing minor wounds; essentially doing gopher work. Interestingly, especially in the VA system, we would reward the patients with cigarettes, which, to this day still amazes me. That we would reward someone in a medical environment with cigarettes seems so unheard of now, but that's the way it was in those days.

The psychiatry rotation was next. As a young person, I walked into a locked ward and met the first patient. He introduced himself as Leroy T. Jenkins, the devil. Needless to say, it was worrisome. Next, I had to try to entice a woman to come out of the bathroom when she had already been shut in there for hours, not willing to talk to anybody or receive any help at all.

We moved on to the rotation of medicine on an open ward with no private rooms. Again, any unwanted work was performed by the interns. Since it was not a pleasant time to be on the wards, we would do almost anything to try to get out of it. One day, my friend and I went to see a test called a pneumoencephalogram, a test I decided right then and there that I would never have any of my patients ever do.

During the test, my friend disappeared to get a drink of water and never came back. The procedure room was next to the emergency room, and when I went to look for him, I found him trying to physically restrain a belligerent, six-foot-four inch tall, ER patient who had been shot in the rectum while jumping a fence attempting to run away from the police. In that moment, well, quite frankly neither man appeared happy to be there.

I jumped in to help and we subdued him while a nurse tried to find something to sedate him. We finally had him down when the chief resident came in and said, "What is going on here?" And the patient said, "Well, I don't know, I don't know. Who is the leader? I will talk to the leader!" To which the chief resident said, "I am the leader. Let him go."

We tried to say this wasn't a good idea, but we did comply.

The patient jumped up and began to strangle the chief resident while exclaiming, "I'm Gamma King of the world. You'll never take me alive!" And the melee started all over again. We were, eventually, able to get him sedated.

Finally the four years of residency was done. It was hard work. At the same time, working emergency room shifts to try and make some money took its toll. Once it was over, it was time to find a job as a physician. My goal was to start my own practice, but at that point I had no money and a lot of debt.

So I decided to join an established practice about two to three hours from home. I knew I had to work to make a living, but I was consistently unhappy in the situation, especially since I was away from home and somewhat homesick.

Looking back, I can identify one reason why I was meant to work at that practice.

This was a story of a young boy who was in the intensive care unit when I met him. At that point, he was in the second week of a severe illness with fever and chills. He was going downhill despite antibiotic therapy and supportive care. He was doing very poorly and I happened to have just completed an infectious disease rotation. I was young and new to the field so I had the time to spend with my patient and his parents. And so I did. I found out that the boy was out in the fields and his father told me he had been bitten by a tick. Lyme disease was relatively new at the time, but I told my senior physician that I felt this was the diagnosis. He disagreed and said that there was no rash. The rash was, at that time, an integral part of the diagnosis. However, as fate would have it, the next day the boy broke out with the typical rash. We changed the antibiotic and the boy did well. His father worked for a newspaper, so we had some wonderful acclaim. It was a wonderful feeling having helped this child, but I knew that it was time for me to return home.

Since I had missed my family, I came back home. However, I still needed some capital. I went to the bank and got an unsecured loan. With that, I started my own practice.

Those were slower times, and again, many sleepless nights, because although I now had a medical degree and a book of knowledge, no one ever taught us about the financial aspects of starting and running a practice. And at first it was almost overwhelming with malpractice insurances and rent, trying to get a staff, trying to buy equipment, and at the same time trying to find patients so that I could make a living.

Fortunately for me, my sister had worked in a physician's office and agreed to help me to start the business. My sister volunteered at first, but I was able to pay her with some time. On the side, I worked at another, already-established practice to get a salary and invest into my new practice. It was there that I met my future wife.

Over the years, with the help of my sister, my wife, and other friends and family members, I was able to acquire a number of different staff members until I had a core of dedicated, loyal, bright, wonderful people who helped the practice grow. I always tried to treat them well, not only because it was the right thing to do, but also because they were a big asset, and I knew it.

The only reason why I felt I had gone to the first practice was to save that boy. And now, I started my own practice in my hometown. I gained hospital privileges. I rented a part-time office. I worked on the side in that established practice to help make some revenue. I also did some ER shifts. And I treated patients everywhere I went.

I had a patient who I admitted to the hospital. And one of the major players at the hospital, the head of a major group, came up and introduced himself to me. He told me they did business theories and if I would refer patients to him, they would refer patients to me. I looked at him and nodded and said, okay. But I actually thought to myself that, instead, I was going to take one patient, give them good care, and they would bring me two patients. Those two would bring me four, et cetera. To me, word of mouth was probably the best marketing and then I wouldn't be dependent on other groups for a living. This is the way my practice grew. Looking back, it was probably the most pleasant time to practice medicine.

I could spend all the time I wanted with each patient. We had a wide variety of people who started to come to us. We had nuns and prostitutes. We had gangsters and federal agents. We had celebrities. No matter who they were or why they came to see me, we always tried to treat each person with dignity and respect. During that time, we built up a fair friendship with all our patients. As the practice got busier, it became more and more difficult to spend a large amount of time with each patient. Throughout my practice, we always tried to continue that, even with starting hospital rounds at 6am, office hours at 9am, going back to the hospital for rounds after 7pm, the days got longer and longer. Regardless, we tried to treat all our patients in the best possible way.

More and more people came to the practice. The patients sometimes would wait long periods of time, but no one complained, or, rather, very few complained, because they realized that when it was their turn, they would also have all the time they needed to talk, to give me their problems, and for us to try to find a solution together.

Then came an interesting turn of events. Insurance companies started to get involved in medical care, and at first, they would approach the physician and promise some patients for a discounted fee. This wasn't a favorable concept, but as time progressed, because the premiums became less costly for the patients, employers would basically make deals with the insurance companies. Insurance policies for health care became more and more popular. There was a discounted fee for each patient and they would cover a panel per patient per month, but with the caveat that now the medical community had to see more patients in a shorter period of time.

I would like to bring you along for this 50 year career so you can understand the system better: where it started, where it is today, and where it is going. By better understanding the system, my hope is you will be able to negotiate it better. I would also like to give you a feeling for the evolution of medicine. Our grandparents had no idea that TVs, microwaves, cars, computers would be everyday events, but society has been transformed by new technology. Likewise, science went from bloodletting, leeches, and home remedies to an understanding of Mendelian genetics, cell theory, and DNA technology. Now we are in the advent of supercomputers, AI, and an understanding of genetic code. Our future is about to change again. As most things in life, when used for good, these advances are a boon for mankind. When used inappropriately, we've seen how dire consequences can be for generations to come..

OVERVIEW

I've learned much from patients over the past 50 years. And I've had many of the same questions from patients recur throughout the years. I want to try to clarify confusion to help patients negotiate the health system better. I give the reader guidance on how to approach the system, how to advocate for themselves, what some of the issues and problems are in health care, and then approach different topics of interest.

There are a number of concepts that will continue throughout the entire book and they are:

-Medicine is both an art and a science to some extent

-Every issue in medicine comes down to this for the patient:

A.) What is the benefit to me?

B.) What is the risk to me?

-Healthcare has become run by corporations and they are dependent on

making profit to stay alive

-No one is perfect.

-The best kind of medicine is preventive medicine.

-Treatment should always be evaluated and benefit your health.

-There's a time to fight and there's a time to realize that it's okay to die.

I've learned from patients that it is not easy to negotiate the system. There are many questions that recur time and time again. I will try to answer some of the questions in this book, along with ways to take care of yourself in a complicated healthcare system, approach and understand the system, how to receive proper care, what some of the prominent issues in healthcare actually are, and help you stay current with what's happening in medicine today.

As I said, for many years, it was a fun time in our practice. We had a diverse waiting room and anyone and everyone would come into the office for all sorts of medical needs. We always insisted that everyone be treated with dignity and respect.

And also that respect was reciprocated. We insisted our staff was respected if a patient wanted to stay in the practice. Once insurance companies started getting into medicine, they decided they would give patients to us for a discounted price. The idea grew more and more and insurance companies became more and more powerful. Ultimately, private practice was about to die, for the most part anyway, because keeping up with malpractice insurance, computerization, staff salaries, benefits, rent, and more meant it was almost impossible to continue the same way of doing business.

Essentially, the hospital systems started to take care of the business part and hired physicians as salaried employees. With that came certain expectations, including time limitations for each patient and each physician.

The physician's salary became dependent on not only the quality of care that a physician provides, but also how many people they see, what the survey feedback said, and how many quality parameters they hit. Although some of this turned out to be for the good, some of it has become challenging, and all of it changed the tenure of medicine.

So in preparing for a visit to your physician, it is helpful for modern patients to understand they have probably 15 to 20 minutes for their doctor to: Listen to you, examine you, make a diagnosis, discuss the problem, and formulate a treatment plan with you. As well as enter all this information into the record. When a patient shows up 15 minutes late, we now only have 5 minutes with the physician to do all these things because there's another patient waiting. It is no longer up to the physician how much time they spend, who they see, or when they see them. It is all computerized and done by the hospital or insurance system. This is done because the health system needs to be viable and make money to survive.

The evolution worsened. As expenses went up with rents, insurances, staff fees, it became more and more difficult to make any profit. I've always felt it was very important to take good care of my staff.

I was blessed over the years of weaning out a lot of deadbeats and ended up with a great crew and always knew they were a wonderful asset. I always tried to treat them well, not only because it was the right thing to do, but because I realized what a great blessing they were to me and the practice. However, as expenses went up, computerization came in. Then insurance companies and the government were requiring electronic medical records, which again was a tremendous cost.

Now hospital systems and insurance companies started to run the health industry, hiring physicians who are salary dependent not only on quality of care issues but also the amount of people seen and feedback from the patients for such things as wait time. So fast forward to the present time, where your average visit is between 15 and 20 minutes per patient.

This is, understandably, somewhat challenging for both the medical team and the patient.

So, what can the patient do to help their own situation?

- Firstly, if you're an early bird, it's best to try to get an early appointment because, if each patient puts the doctor five minutes behind and you're the tenth person in line, you're now 15 minutes waiting in a waiting room.
- Secondly, be on time. If you have a 20-minute allotted slot and you're 15 minutes late for your appointment, that means you now have five minutes to try to tell the physician what your needs are.
- Thirdly, write down your problems so that you don't forget, when you are there to see your physician, all the issues that you want to discuss.
- Fourthly, write down your medications and dosages.

I had a delightful patient, a little old woman, who I had asked to write her medications down to bring to her next visit so I could review them. To her credit, she did. She wrote, "A.M., one o'clock in the morning: one blue pill, one red pill; lunch time: one red pill; dinner time: one blue pill, one red pill. Stop, start again." This was not what I had hoped for or expected and, while adorable, it wasn't very helpful.

But if you write down your medication(s) and dosage(s) and any refills that you need, this will help speed your visit along, make sure your chart is accurate, and ensure your needs are met.

Once you discuss your problems with the physician and a diagnosis is made, this diagnosis should be discussed. Additionally, you'll want to know what the game plan looks like going forward. There should be shared decision making in which way you wish to approach a problem. Let me say at this point, that any physician, any *good* physician, should never complain about a patient obtaining a second opinion somewhere else, especially regarding a serious diagnosis.

Physicians each look at things differently and what one person may think warrants surgery, another may think should be treated with medication. Your physician should be able to tell you what the treatment is, why they recommend it, what the problem is with not following recommendations, what the side effects are, and if you're in agreement with the treatment plan. ‘

If you are not in agreement, then I would seek a second opinion with a qualified specialist to see if they agree with that treatment plan.

One of the comments patients often say to me is, “Well, this medication has side effects.” Understanding that anything you put in your body has a potential for side effects is a good starting point to evaluate the benefit versus the risk. **The question is *always*, does the benefit** of you taking that medication, or does the benefit of you getting that procedure, the benefit of you getting that test performed, **outweigh the risk** to you otherwise? If it makes sense, then doing that makes sense. Because we should keep in mind that the disease process also has side effects. Many times the side effects to the disease are much worse than any potential side effects of the medicine used to treat it.

The other caution I give to patients is to be leery of testing in facilities in which the referring physician has a financial interest. I'm not saying that there's anything underhanded at work, but again, stay vigilant. Sometimes these tests are not necessary to make a diagnosis or treatment, but rather to make profit. An important question to ask is, “How would this test, how would this procedure, how would this surgery, how would this medication benefit me and my quality of life moving forward?

This is especially true with some surgical procedures. Patients have said to me, “Oh, [this or that person, physician] is knife happy.” But the fact of the matter is, there is most often no mal-intent in the recommendation. It is the way a surgeon looks at things. Other disciplines may look at treatment options differently.

And this is where you, as the patient, can do your homework. Be prepared to talk to your primary care physician about the various options available to you.

Once a treatment plan is recommended, you should be aware of the positive effect and the negative effect of such treatment, whether it be taking an aspirin or undergoing significant surgery. Patients often say to me, my drug has side effects. My answer to them is, “So does the disease process.”

Always remember the question you should be asking is, does the benefit of me taking this pill outweigh the risk of me having a serious medical complication that may debilitate me?

Chapter 1

Suppose for a moment that you're ready for your office visit, you've gone in, you have a diagnosis, you have a treatment plan, you're happy with the visit. However, now it's time to pay for your care.

Some patients are self-pay, which means they do not have insurance, insurance will not cover a particular type of exam/diagnostic/treatment, or they choose to pay out-of-pocket for certain medical expenses. Most people opt for insurance coverage, when they can, so let's take a look at insurances.

Many people have insurance through their employers. Some patients are able to choose, some have government-backed plans, and the others may have Medicare or Medicaid. And there are plenty of other insurances. A patient of mine once said to me "Well, you know, doctor, there are no free lunches," when she went to a HMO seminar and her lunch was provided. No truer words were spoken.

If you're able to decide on an insurance plan, your decisions are probably going to be very different if you are a young, healthy individual versus an elderly, debilitated patient. Each insurance has certain rules and regulations. Some premiums are less, however, when you go to use them, not everything you'd like done may be covered.

Some medications you take may not be covered. Certain hospital systems may not be covered. Certain office visits, procedures, and/or testing may not be covered. These are items you should consider before choosing a policy.

Also, investigate the amount of items you can cover. There is often out-of-pocket money you will be required to pay. Therefore, if you use the health system regularly and you opt for low premium insurance, you may find yourself paying much more over the year in deductibles, co-pays, and out-of-pocket expenses. It helps to know ahead of time what you will pay for emergency room visits versus urgent care and hospital stays. Is there a limit to the out-of-pocket that you would have to pay in a year? These are important questions you want to ask before you commit to a policy.

Medicare is unique in that patients over 65 can get hospital coverage and then can also elect a supplement plan. Since the hospital coverage pays 80% of hospital stays, and may or may not pay certain amounts for visits and procedures, the supplement plan would take up the remainder and the additional 20% that's not paid by Medicare in the hospital. Please note that nursing home insurance is altogether different and usually separate policies are required.

Hospice should be covered by most plans, but again, it's good to check with the agent before you make a decision.

Chapter 2

While I was doing hospital work, I had an interesting revelation. We had a patient, an elderly female, who was having a heart attack. TPK had just come out and been approved at that time. She was literally dying in front of us. We had given her IV nitro, morphine, beta blockers, IV fluids. She had crushing chest pain and EKG changes despite the regimen. She was seriously ill. We administered TPA and it was amazing. The patient's EKG normalized. She felt better. The pain went away, and she did well. We received some accolades after that, but I thought to myself, *well, if I'm doing such a good job,* ***why*** *is my patient in the intensive care unit in the first place?*

So we decided to change the tenure of the practice to try to educate our patients on risk factors and how to keep them out of the hospital. We placed a special emphasis on how to especially keep out of the ICU.

Obviously there is a genetic component to disease, which, at the present time, we only have limited ability to evaluate and/or manipulate genes. But this will be a treatment plan in the future. There are factors that are under our control. I'd like to cover these in more depth.

First of all, I would advise a yearly exam with your primary care physician, a complete blood, and urine analysis. These help to isolate any problems you, as an individual, may have and should begin to work on in a proactive manner. A routine blood panel is a very cost-effective way to screen for side effects and can give us a wealth of information. In this way, we can look at the components of your bone marrow, measure blood sugar and cholesterol, as well as evaluate kidney and liver functions, electrolytes counts, and check for protein in the urine.

The more common problems that I see in my office every day have to do with: Hypertension, Hyperlipidemia, Diabetes, Infectious diseases, Weight reduction, Anxiety, Depression, Cardiac issues, Rheumatoid issues, and Cancers. I may also see a variety of other issues. Most of these are picked up with screening tools. These tools are usually age adjusted. Since many cancers occur over the age of 50, you'll see additional blood tests, like a PSA, performed. Procedures such as colonoscopy, EKG, and chest x-ray done and mammograms are also commonly recommended in the elderly population.

Aside from genetic components, I'd like to review some of these problems now. Some are grouped together, as it can be difficult to cover all the different issues that affect overall health.

Chapter 3

Hypertension, or high blood pressure, is excessive pressure against the vessel walls. This is a major cause of morbidity and mortality worldwide and a very common reason for patient visits to my office.

Blood pressure readings should remain below 140 over 90. If you have other conditions, like diabetes, heart disease, kidney disease, keeping it below 130 over 80 is preferable. The reason why you want to keep your blood pressure low is to protect your heart, eye, kidney, and prevent neurological damages as a result of injury to the vessel wall. Symptoms may be dizziness, chest pain, nosebleeds, neurological deficits, headaches, and in the worst conditions, heart attack, stroke, or kidney failure. Causes of hypertension may include a genetic component, hormonal component, changes in kidney and vessel walls due to arteriosclerosis, and/or sleep apnea.

There are a number of factors which can aggravate hypertension, including increased salt intake, obesity, alcoholism, cigarette smoking, lack of exercise, with a high sodium diet probably being the worst offender.

So if you've been diagnosed with hypertension, what are some of the things that you can do? Well, probably the best thing is a low-sodium diet. Sodium is probably the major culprit in elevating a patient's blood pressure numbers. Secondly, consider stress management. Yoga and prayer are helpful in this manner since anxiety can, at least, cause short-term elevations in blood pressure. Physical activity is helpful, weight reduction, and decreasing alcohol and/or smoking are all helpful in lowering blood pressure values. Certain herbs such as cinnamon, garlic, basil, parsley, celery seed, thyme, ginger are also beneficial.

If blood pressure continues to remain elevated, then in the office we usually recommend some pharmacological agent. The different agents include beta blockers, ACE inhibitors, ARBs, calcium channel blockers, diuretics, and central acting agents. Usually we try to tailor the treatment medication to the patient.

For example, if the patient has migraines and hypertension, a beta blocker is helpful in treating both. If the patient has diabetes, an ACE or an ARB agent is helpful to protect the kidneys against the effects of diabetes in addition to lowering blood pressure. Special conditions, such as pregnancy, limit certain medications. Usually labetalol, hydralazine, alpha-methyldopa, and nifedipine are safe agents in pregnancy.

00:00:01

Herbals include cardamom, C-A-R-D-A-M-O-M, Chinese, cat's claw, bacope,

monarium, B-E-C-O-P-A-M-O-N-N-I-E-N-I, benixi, benaha, tihatang,

B-A-N-X-I-A-B-A-I-Z-H-A-T-I-A-N-A-T-A-N-G.

00:00:40

In terms of drinks, black and green tea, beet juice, pomegranate juice, and skim milk

may be helpful.

Chapter 4

GI symptoms are a common cause of both hospital and office visits. Patients with more serious problems, such as pancreatitis, cirrhosis, hepatitis, diverticulitis, GI bleeds may end up as a hospital admission.

Most office visits consist of symptoms of either gerd, abdominal pain, ulcer disease, nausea, vomiting and/or diarrhea. Unexplained anemia in adults and/or unexplained weight loss requires a full workup, including GI studies like radiology, endoscopy, or colonoscopy.

As far as prevention goes, what can you do to protect yourself against some of these problems? Alcohol, excessive caffeine, stress, non-steroidal anti-inflammatory medications, such as Motrin, may all play a part in the etiology of these diseases. Excessive alcohol can often lead to pancreatitis, gastritis, and cirrhosis. Spicy foods may play a part. Elevating the head of the bed, not eating late at night, limiting spicy foods, caffeine, and alcohol also help alleviate GERD symptoms.

Hepatitis may be spread by blood-borne infections, so hand-washing is important. Stress management is helpful through activities such as prayer, tai chi, yoga, and exercise. All these may help.

If you do have diverticulitis, avoid nuts and seeds in your diet. As far as hepatitis, it can also be spread by needle sticks and bodily fluids, so condom use with sexual contact is important. Tattoos should only be given by tattoo artists who adhere to the utmost cleanliness standards.Steps, such as drug addicts not sharing needles, help prevent spreading disease

There are many causes of diarrheal disease. Some related to travel. Some related to swimming in non-chlorinated or salt water. Improper food preparation is a major cause of diarrhea.

When preparing food, remember to make sure that the food is cooked properly. Ensure that items such as turkey or pork reach an adequate temperature. After eating, do not place the food in a previous surface area that may have been contaminated before eating it. These surfaces include places like countertops, table surfaces, and refrigerator shelves.

Viral gastroenteritis can be quite severe, but will usually self-eliminate within a day or so. The key is to not get dehydrated and not to eat until symptoms are better. Self-care includes a BRAT diet, a mixture of bananas and rice are helpful in slowing the stool down, and if medication is needed to slow the gut, take it sparingly and do not eat if you take an excessive amount of medication then, once the acute episode passes, you'll find yourself constipated.

Herbs that may help the GI tract include licorice, cat's claw, chamomile, dandelion, juniper, and peppermint. Medications include antacids, acid blockers, antimotility agents, and proton pump inhibitors.

Chapter 5

Let's now look at some of the factors that are under your control in trying to live a long, healthy life. I want to start by explaining that many of these factors are interrelated and some are causative. We all have certain cues in our life that set off our behaviors. Whether it be stress, boredom, excitement, et cetera, we may react many times without thinking.

The psychiatry people call this automaticity. You look at that piece of apple pie and eat it without thinking about it at all, or light that cigarette after your coffee without acknowledging the detrimental effects. Afterwards, the person may feel guilt thinking back upon what they did.

Part of understanding your behavior is to start to recognize the cue. Once you recognize the cue, whether it be anxiety, or any other issue, you can work on changing the behavior. Modifying risk factors is very important in your overall health and in keeping you out of the hospital or intensive care unit. Moving one's hands to mouth, known as oral gratification, is a very comforting motion in humans. So again, if you think about smoking, drinking, and drugs, many times these are hand-to-mouth comforters. With that in mind, let's look at some of the problems that we see in the office every day and how we can work on preventing little problems from becoming larger ones.

Chapter 6

Type II Diabetes is the cause of some of my sickest chronically debilitated patients. Diabetes mellitus is a condition in which there is too much sugar in the blood. It develops when your pancreas does not make enough insulin or your body cannot utilize the insulin effectively. Sugar comes into the diet predominantly from carbohydrates.

The diabetic symptoms of polydipsia, drink too much, polyphagia, eat too much, polyurea, urinating too much, can be present when blood sugar is out of control. Most subtle problems, however, include altered immune responses resulting in infections, including fungal infections, and also visual disturbances. Causes include a genetic component, autoimmune issues, obesity, lack of exercise, diet, hormonal imbalances, and certain medications, along with pancreatic damage.

Diabetes can cause acute problems, such as diabetic-related ketoacidosis, which is an acid-based disease, eye, kidney, neurological, skin, sexual dysfunction, gastroparesis, and even complications as drastic as amputations. The first step in treatment is diet and exercise. I have seen tremendous improvement in patients who stick to a strict low carbohydrate diet, exercise, and have lost a significant amount of weight. Prevention begins by not automatically eating high carbohydrates mindlessly, but to be aware of what you're doing before you do it.

Awareness is the key. Ideally, we want to keep little problems, little problems. The goal is to try to prevent big problems that are within our control.

Suppose you're an anxious person, or something in your environment triggers you, and you automatically start eating high processed foods. They can lead to diabetes, which then leads to complications, some of which may end you up in ICU, and some of which may give you a chronic, debilitating lifestyle. I've often told my patients that I don't want them to say that if they had known a better physician who explained what was happening to them, and that they had the power to alter their course, that they would not be in intensive care at that point.

After diet and exercise, herbal treatments are available which can help manage symptoms. These include cinnamon, aloe, ginseng, stevia, and dandelion. There are numerous medications for the treatment of diabetes, including insulin, there are older agents and newer products. What most do is help the insulin secrete pancreas, affect the liver, help for better peripheral utilization of the sugar, or eliminate sugar from the body.

I'd like to also address high cholesterol and diabetes. Cholesterol is a fatty substance in your blood. There's good cholesterol that the body uses for healthy cell function, but there is also a bad type of cholesterol, which is atherogenic and is a major cause of agent in the development of vessel disease. Causes include such things as genetic components and a diet high in high fat processed foods.

Actively working to lower your cholesterol is an attempt to stop progression of heart attack, stroke, and/or peripheral vascular disease. After diet and exercise, herbal remedies include red yeast rice, niacin, bile salts, soy, hawthorn, garlic, and fish oils. Drug management includes classes of drugs known as statins also known as HMG-CoA reductase inhibitors and PCSK9 inhibitors also known as proprotein convertase subtilisin/kexin type-9 inhibitors.

Again, controlling the urge to eat outside hunger, smoke, drink and/or take drugs can pay dividends for your health in the long term.

Chapter 7

Once you're at the visit, and various suggestions are made, it's important to understand why the test is being done, and what is going to be done with the information that you're going to be given. For example, I have people who have said that they would never have cardiac bypass surgery, no matter the reason. This is perfectly reasonable, however, if that's the case, then my question is, "Why, then, go through a catheterization, or calcium scoring, or an exercise stress test? The testing should be focused on what the treatment plan would be."

Along those lines, I was once asked to do a consultation for a family member of one of my patients who is severely ill in a nursing home. Although I did not really wish to do it, she was a good patient and was concerned about her elderly aunt. When I did the consult, it was clear to me that the patient was going in the direction of sepsis. She was an elderly woman, with dementia, who did not recognize anyone, on the verge of multiple organ failure, with a gangrenous leg. The recommendations were that she have surgery for an amputation of her leg. My advice to her niece was not to do the surgery. Her response back to me was that her aunt would die. And my answer was, "Yes, she will." To what end should we continue to torture this woman with her very poor quality of life who is on death's bed even with amputating her leg. Would it improve her quality of life or change her outcome? While it was certainly a hard reality to accept that she would die, it was better than watching her suffer first and die anyway.

This was a difficult decision, but once the family and I discussed the patient's multiple organ failures, dementia, and sepsis, all were in agreement. But these types of decisions are personal and not always clear-cut.

And so many health care institutions have ethics committees who address issues, issues which may arrive in patient care. The committee is usually made up of medical and non-medical people, including lay people. In general, medical ethics committees provide a framework for moral judgments for individual patients.

There are four principles usually accepted in medical ethics, and that is autonomy, which is respect for the patient's rights to make their own self-determination, beneficence duty to do good for the patient, non malfeasance, do no harm, and justice to treat each patient equally and fairly. Ideally all these principles should always be followed by all of an individual's health care team.

We will look at terminal processes and hospice care at greater depth later in the book.

Chapter 8

Many patients come to the office with musculoskeletal complaints of pain, stiffness, tenderness, swelling and deformity of a joint or muscle pain. Causes can include wear and tear on the joint, poor body mechanics, previous trauma, and certain highly processed foods.

Risk factors include age and family history, previous injury to the joint, and obesity. The most logical reason to treat is because if pain worsens over time, the joint becomes destroyed and it becomes more difficult to do everyday chores. I like to look at arthritis in one or two categories. Either wear and tear type arthritis or inflammatory. Dyskinetic, disease, hip, knee problems. Carpal tunnel examples of degenerative changes, rheumatoid arthritis, lupus gout are examples of inflammation. There are many others, but these are the most commonly seen. Changes may occur in the back knee, and may radiate down the extremities. Inflammatory arthritis is usually bilateral, smaller joints, and much more inflammatory in nature. Gout usually presents as a very painful, isolated joint with most arthritic conditions. I traditionally take a conservative position and only recommend surgery as a last resort. If there's neurological impingement prior to surgical correction, then a second opinion would always be helpful. Our first line of therapy is ice immobilized injuries followed by physical therapy and gradually moving to weighted exercise. Joint injections are often helpful. Most conditions will improve with rest and time. Tylenol and non-steroidals like Motrin and naproxen are helpful for relieving inflammation, but long-term use may affect the kidney and/or GI tract. Steroids are very helpful with acute inflammation, but can also have long-term side effects and they should also be tapered. Alternative and herbal treatments include chondroitin, glucosamine, MSM, turmeric, butterbur, dandelion, wintergreen, casserole ginger, licorice, parsley, and kelp. Massage and chiropractic care are both helpful and I have also seen good results with acupuncture in patients with nerve pain.

Chapter 9

Let's consider another disorder we can change. COPD is defined as a group of lung diseases which make it difficult to breathe. It is a chronic inflammatory lung condition. Although there are some genetic and environmental factors, the major cause is cigarette smoking. Illustrating its addiction, we have had many patients trying to smoke through their tracheostomy tube.

As you age, you want to be able to walk at least short distances without struggling to breathe and nothing upsets me more than seeing one of my patients on a ventilator. By stopping smoking at any age, you can salvage lung tissue. If you recognize the cue, whether it be caffeine, boredom, aggravation, excitement, and once you recognize it, change the behavior, your lungs will thank you.

Some useful herbal treatments for breathing include Butterbur, Juniper, Eucalyptus, Flax, Marshmallow, Ashwagandha, and Rosemary.

Medications include a various number of inhalers, Singulair, oral steroids, and there are some newer agents as well.

Chapter 10

Among the most common visits in the office are related to anxiety and mood disorders. Anxiety is concerned over many aspects of your life. Stress in itself is not inherently bad. Stress has a purpose in defending a person against threats. But if that level of worry escalates, problems arise, which affect the person, their day-to-day functioning, and may become overwhelming.

Likewise, depression is defined as a loan of the patient's mood. Again, if it progresses, it can cause a loss of the other activities. Depression can be the underlying cause of a number of medical problems. Reacting to loss, anger, hormonal changes can precipitate mental discord, drug abuse, other addictions, self-isolation, social isolation, inability to perform daily functions, and could lead to suicide ideation if it worsens. Primarily, one must recognize that depression is the underlying cause.

I've had patients who've come in arguing with one another because the husband said his wife gave him a salad for lunch and dinner the night before. I'm sure we can agree they are not actually arguing about the salads. Or let's consider a young person who's undergoing hormonal changes and has no idea why they feel so down. Others who've had a significant loss or disability.

The key to it is not succumbing to automatic behavior secondary to the cue but rather finding some healthy alternative. Many patients successfully use techniques such as meditation, tai chi, prayer, and yoga to help them through tough times. I have many times asked patients to take their negative energy and direct it to something helpful and useful.

The cause is usually, again, some genetic predisposition, neurotransmitter disruption, and environmental factors and how they affect the brain. There is some thought that a trigger for the activation of the neuronal circuit in those areas, is an abnormal sensitivity to disturbance of acid-base balance in the brainstem.

Feeling nervous, trouble sleeping, GI symptoms, feeling down, more we believe in these substances at first. Agoraphobia, social anxiety, panic disorder, separation anxiety, substance abuse, anxiety, and depression, all appear in the same church. But when tolerance and addiction follow, your health is in serious danger.

Some useful herbal therapy for anxiety include valerian, skullcap, rhodiola, r-h-o-d-i-o-l-a, passionflower, lemon balm, java, hops, chamomile, bacopa, b-a-c-o-p-a, a-s-h-w-a-g-a-n-d-h-a. In terms of medical treatment, there are benzodiazepine, serotonin reuptakes, and some of the older agents. They have a calming or a depressive effect.

Herbs that help treat depression are black cohosh, rhodiolola and St. John's wort. There are a number of medications used to treat depression, many of which work on the neurotransmitters. The most common are serotonin reuptakes.

Causes in both these conditions include genetics which play a significant role, as there are higher incidences in families, along with environmental factors and neurotransmitters. Substances that are shown to be panicogenic, include sodium lactate, inhalation of carbon dioxide, cystokinin, tetrapeptide, caffeine, yohirumine, y-o-h-i-m-i-n-e-t-e-t-r-a-p-t-i-d-e-c-a-f-f-e-n-e-c-a-f-e-n-e-c-a- B-I-N-E, isoprotonol, I-S-O-P-R-O-T-E-R-N-O-L, and the benzodiazepine antagonist, F-L-U-M-A-Z-E-N-I-L. Functional MRI studies show certain areas of the brain are infected.

Chapter 11

A word about substance abuse, including drugs and alcohol:

The recreational user can turn it off or on. The addicted user cannot. The problem either way is that these activities build up tolerance and addiction, which can cause many health problems.

The complexity of the issue goes even further. We have largely seen and are aware of the medical and social issues that have arisen from addictive persons, patients, various sexual diseases, violence, lack of social skills, cirrhosis, encephalopathy, ascites neuropathy, to name a few that we see in everyday practice. Unfortunately, like many disease processes, some patients are in denial and continue their automatic behavior. They do not, or can not, stop and think of what effects the addiction has on their health and also the toll that is taken on by their loved ones. Over the years, I've also come to conclude that the only one that can stop a patient's addiction is the actual patient themself.

No matter how well-meaning, loving, and strong a family may be, a loved one may be, a significant other may be, unless the patient wants to change, it will not happen. And the results sometimes can be devastating, but as I tell our patients, it is not a one-size-fits-all.

That is that person's choice. You do not have the right to tell them how to live. On the other hand, they do not have the right to bring you down with them. So if a patient is willing to get help, the family should be supportive and do everything they can to help them. If they're not, the family should disengage. This is usually a difficult concept to achieve.

Chapter 12

00:00:02
We have reviewed a number of risk factors, many of which are related to heart disease and stroke. By recognizing some of these factors, you are able to influence both conditions. Heart disease comes in many different forms. Many patients come to the office with coronary artery disease, which can tend to cause heart attacks and unfortunate progressive congestive heart failure. Other patients can present with abnormal rhythms, infiltrative disease, valvular disease, or.
00:00:37
pericardial disease. Of course, the treatment varies with the different types and medications pacemakers are sometimes needed. But the first recommendation is lifestyle change, controlling blood pressure, sugar, cholesterol, stop smoking, and limiting alcoholConsumption, along with avoiding stimulants, less salt, exercise, and taking prescribed.
00:01:09
medications are all important factors. Heart disease can be managed effectively with lifestyle change, medications, and sometimes surgical procedures. Herbs use for healthy heart include Astragal, Redix, Tongyinluo.
00:01:52
. Heart healthy spices include turmeric, garlic, black pepper. In terms of vitamins C, K, D, E, B3 or niacin are helpful. Green tea is also thought to be helpful.
00:02:24
As always, check with your physician prior to taking any supplements.

Chapter 13

It is my belief that these two conditions are indirectly significant etiological factors, and many other disease disorders which are treated in the office. As I previously said, the hand-to-mouth motion is very comforting for humans. Eating, drinking, smoking, drugs happen daily.

What happens when these become excessive and out of control? And why does it happen? It goes back to cues. There are cues to eat, drink, smoke, and take drugs. In excess, these are all very detrimental to the body's overall health. One was a smoker who smoked four packs a day. One was a drinker who had a bottle of scotch each night. One was a drug addict who had their parents lose their house. And one was a male who told me he masturbated six to eight times a day. It is important to note that this is not because these patients found this enjoyable. Engaging in such activities leaves little time for anything else pleasurable in life.

Once we really look at why they are doing it, patients are able to recognize what sets them off, and ultimately change their behavior. If these patients had continued the way they were going, they would have ended up with significant morbidity and mortality.

Smoking is also a major contributing factor in the development of heart attack and stroke. Coronary artery disease is one of the major causes of death worldwide, but even more disturbing, is seeing our patients struggling to deal with even everyday routine activities. A low-fat diet, exercise, controlling diabetes, managing hypertension, lowering cholesterol, and addressing inflammation are determining factors in decreasing progressions of disease.

Chapter 14

The next group of visits I would like to talk about fall into the infectious categories. Upper respiratory infections, coughs, sinusitis, bronchitis, influenza, COVID, ear infections, are relatively common occurrences. Most times the cause of the agent is viral and antibiotics are not helpful, and as a matter of fact, may be harmful. There are some antiviral medications that can be used, but for the most part, the viral symptoms will resolve with conservative care.

A common bacterial agent that *should* be treated with antibiotics is strep since these can lead to complications later down the line, such as heart and kidney disease. With the advent of a rapid stress test in the office, this can be quickly diagnosed. There is also point-of-care testing in the office for influenza and COVID.

Pneumonia is a more serious problem with symptoms of fever, chills, cough, shortness of breath, and sometimes coughing up blood.

Hearing a muffled area on an auscultation, through a stethoscope, during physical exam and an interpretation of a chest x-ray may be the way to make a diagnosis and distinguish it also from other conditions such as tuberculosis or a malignant infiltrate. Sometimes a CAT scan is indicated to make the diagnosis.

So what are some of the things you can do for prevention? One of the most important concepts is proper hand washing with soap and water. Also, it would be prudent to keep away from crowds in times of epidemics, especially areas where there is yelling, singing, screaming. Proper rest and nutrition and antioxidants may be helpful with enhancing the immune response.

Urinary tract infection is a common office visit that we see, especially in female patients. Since the urethra is small, it's easy to introduce infection with improper stool wiping, hot tub use, intercourse, etc. Symptoms include urinary frequency burning. In the office, there's a point of service testing again, which can give an indication, but the actual diagnosis is made by urine culture. If it seems that the urine is contaminated, however, treatment should start, depending on the culture, and should really take 48 hours to obtain the result. In men with urinary infections one must consider some type of obstruction and a urologist should be consulted.

Some of the most common infections worldwide include syphilis, gonorrhea, HIV, HPV, chlamydia, herpes, molluscum, hepatitis B, mycoplasma, giardia, haemophilus, and cytomegalovirus. Symptoms may include urethritis, discharge, swollen lymph nodes, pelvic inflammatory disease, ulcerations, warts, lice, scabies, or intestinal infections. Prevention includes limiting sexual contacts, condom use, prophylaxis exposure regimens, immunization, and routine testing for gonorrhea, HIV, and syphilis. If treatment is needed, it is always important to complete the entire course of therapy.

Amongst some of the most difficult patients to diagnose are patients who have come back from traveling outside the country. In addition, with the influx of new immigrants into the United States, we're seeing an increase in certain types of diseases. Diseases such as dengue, Amoebiasis tuberculosis, giardia, chikungunya cholera, schistosomiasis, typhoid, yellow fever, rabies, syphilis, brucellosis, tuberculosis, shigellosis travels diarrhea, are a few examples of differentials we acquire when looking at a patient's symptoms and travel history.

The description diagnosis and treatment of these conditions are beyond the scope of this book and and could be the subject of an additional book. My focus is to inform you how to keep yourself safe against dealing with these unpleasant, sometimes fatal, often preventable, diseases.

With rural travel to places outside of the United States, there are a number of ways to become infected with a variety of diseases. You can contact disease by water, food, animal contact, soil, vectors such as insects, bites, and sexual contact. In terms of prevention, this is a strong area where immunization can be very helpful. There are immunizations against yellow fever, typhus, rabies, meningococcus, cholera, hepatitis A, and Japanese encephalitis. A chemoprophylaxis vaccination is recommended for certain endemic areas.

The CDC has a valuable website for travelers, and has a section called Travelers Clinic, which gives information on epidemiology of the area, travel, threats of various countries, and other pertinent area information.

In general, the United States, Europe, Canada, New Zealand, and Australia are relatively safe for travel. Other countries, the risk of acquiring an infectious disease depends on where you are going and the length of the time you are staying.

General principles to protect yourself include:

-Avoid swimming in fresh waters in tropical environments

-Meat and fish should be cooked thoroughly and not smoked or salted

-Water should be purified, either boiled or come from a safe source

-Peel skins of fruits and vegetables

-Avoid dairy and lettuce

-Prevent insects bites with netting and insect repellents along with appropriate clothing

-Caution should be given to medication given by pharmacists in a foreign country, as you should understand, what exactly the medication is, where it came from, what it does, and its potential side effects

A special note about COVID-19 infection:

It is caused by a coronavirus called SARS-CoV-2. It mutates like many other viruses, and this is the reason for periodic vaccine updates and boosters. The virus spreads by droplets, and you can get it airborne or by touching an infected area, and then touching your eyes, nose, or mouth. Symptoms range from cold symptoms to serious respiratory illnesses. There may be some loss of taste or smell, which eventually returns. There are tests to help with the diagnosis.

These include a PCR test for the virus and a rapid antigen test, which can be done quickly, to help prevent infection. There are vaccines available. It remains important to avoid crowds during epidemics.

Hand washing is essential and protective gear works as a strategy to try to limit exposure to the infection. Treatment is many times symptomatic and include rest, fluids, self-isolation, and conservative therapy. Monoclonal antibodies are available and there are two antivirals that may be taken, as well. Care must be given with the antivirals, however, because they interact with various other medications and must be carefully adjusted to renal function.

Chapter 15

In addition to infectious diseases that can spread from humans to humans, there are also infections that can be spread from animals to humans in different ways. These include bites, licks, direct contact, ingestion, inhalation, or through vectors, like mosquitoes, fleas, and ticks. Additionally, environmental causes, sexual contact, bacterial viruses, rickettsial parasites, and fungi can be transmitted across species.

Some of the infections seen are Q fever, leptospirosis, salmonellosis leptospirosis, Yersinosis, Lyme's disease, psittacosis, Trichomonas, cat scratch fever, E. coli, Toxoplasmosis, Plague, Encephalitis, Zika, Yellow Fever, just to name a few.

The most common seen in my office practice are Lyme's disease and Salmonellosis. Ticks are the vectors in Lyme's disease, as well as in a number of other diseases, such as Rocky mountain spotted fever. An interesting finding of this last disease is that certain patients who have been bitten by the Lone Star tick, the tick which transmits Rocky-Mountain Spotted fever, develop a meat allergy, known as Alpha-Gal syndrome.

Lyme symptoms usually include fever, headache, myalgia, followed by a rash. Untreated, it can lead to severe complications long term. Salmonella is another common cause for office visits. Chicks, farm animals, reptiles and amphibians, are all potential sources and can result in severe intestinal problems in humans.

Prevention of these problems include avoidance of strange animals and proper handling of carcasses. Sterilizing water that may be contaminated. Having pets treated properly with tick and flea medications. Cooking meats properly to appropriate temperatures.

And most importantly, proper hand washing with soap and water after dealing with animals.

Proper treatment is an important factor. Ideally, amphibians should not be kept as pets in households that have children less than five years old, or pregnant mothers, elderly people, or people who are immunocompromised.

Chapter 16

Vaccines, likewise, are age-appropriate. Whether you take a vaccine or not is both an individual decision and many times also impacts public health. Any elderly person who has suffered from smallpox or polio in the past will attest to how good a vaccination program is, for not only individuals, but for society as a whole. People who have had side effects from vaccines will call them a bane. Again, the question is, as an individual, in your circumstance, does it make sense for you to take the precaution of getting a vaccine?

To bring things up to date, if we use the COVID vaccine as an example, if you are a young healthy person, with no risk factors, and live a healthy lifestyle, I don't know that it makes sense to take a COVID vaccine, since you would probably be able to weather the infection with natural immunity. On the other hand, if you were frail, elderly, a person with risk factors, it makes sense for you to take it because if you get the disease there's a good chance you're going to end up in intensive care with a respiratory issue.

During the peak of the COVID was one of the few times that I thought about leaving medicine since it was a scary time when it first came out. No one knew exactly what we were dealing with. It felt very similar to the beginning of AIDS in the eighties when we were still in the hospital seeing seriously ill people and didn't quite understand the transmission or pathophysiology and had felt the population in general, and potentially each individual, was at significant risk.

Chapter 17

We have reviewed a number of risk factors, many of which are related to heart disease and stroke. By recognizing some of these factors, you are able to influence both conditions. Heart disease comes in many different forms. Many patients come to the office with coronary artery disease, which can tend to cause heart attacks and unfortunate progressive congestive heart failure. Other patients can present with abnormal rhythms, infiltrative disease, valvular disease, or pericardial disease.

Of course, the treatment varies with the different types and medications pacemakers are sometimes needed. But the first recommendation is lifestyle change, controlling blood pressure, sugar, cholesterol, stop smoking, and limiting alcohol consumption, along with avoiding stimulants, less salt, exercise, and taking prescribed medications are all important factors. Heart disease can be managed effectively with lifestyle change, medications, and sometimes surgical procedures. Herbs used for a healthy heart include Astragal, Redix, Tongxinluo.

Heart healthy spices include turmeric, garlic, black pepper. In terms of vitamins C, K, D, E, B3 or niacin are helpful. Green tea is also thought to be helpful.

As always, check with your physician prior to taking any supplements.

Chapter 18

Hospital and office visits will sometimes involve patients struggling with a cancer diagnosis. There are many different types of cancer in different locations. Most of the cause by genetic changes that lead to uncontrolled cell growth. Environmental factors do also play a role,especially items like asbestos, radiation, tobacco, alcohol, toxic substances. Also, diet, vaccines, hormones, and workplace chemicals can be included in environmental contributors.

Symptoms may vary depending on the organ and body part involved. But unexplained fever, weight loss, night sweats, unexplained respiratory symptoms, GI symptoms, lumps, bumps, non-healing lesions, mold changes, should raise red flags and warrant diagnostic evaluation.

Treatment consists of chemotherapy, radiation therapy, surgery, and new models such as immunotherapy, targeted chemotherapy, hormonal modulation, stem cell therapy, and genetic manipulation, along with cancer vaccines.

There are no specific herbal remedies for any cancer, but any of the above supplements, such as ginkgo biloba, pomegranate, rosemary, and willow bark may enhance immunity.

For our purposes, I would like to reinforce prevention. Appropriately recommended testing like mammograms, colon screening, PSA tests, blood markers, skin exams, self-exams, transvaginal ultrasound, and low-dose CT scanning can pay large dividends in the long run to avoid serious, future problems.

Chapter 19

While most of the information in this book is aimed at keeping you alive and healthy, despite everyone's best efforts, death or the cessation of bodily functions occurs. In many cases, it is preceded by terminal or debilitating illness. Some of the most common causes of death in this country are related to cardiovascular events, cancer, and accidents.

Palliative care is a type of medical care that provides comfort and focuses on quality of life for people with serious illness. It can be instituted either at home or at an institution. It usually consists of another of medical disciplines including nursing, physicians, psychologists, social workers, and therapists. It attempts to care for both alleviation of stress and management of physical symptoms. It is usually done at the same time that treatment for the disease is being given.

Unlike hospice care, which is a specialized form of palliative care, focusing on making the terminal patient more comfortable, usually treatment is only symptomatic in hospice care, without aggressive medical management.

Studies have indicated that the last sense to go in a dying patient is hearing, so talking to a dying patient is important. It is difficult as a physician to deal with a dying patient, and it is easy to want to look at this situation as defeat, even though we may have done everything we could to prevent it from happening. Equally disturbing, for me, is dealing with family and friends who have a deep grief and emotional sadness, which is understandable due to this loss in their life.

I try to focus on the good memories of the patient and find it to be helpful and comforting to myself and the family. I want to add that I believe, in the past 50 years, when dealing with dying patients, I've heard regrets in terms of relationships, things that could have been done during their life that weren't, things for which people were remorseful; but, not once in 50 years have I heard a patient say that they wish they had a bigger car, a boat, a second home, or material possession. This always helps keep things in perspective for me.

Chapter 20

If you find yourself going into the hospital, it is very important that you have family or friends support to help interpret and guide you in some decision making.

The same is true for nursing homes. Many times things can be overlooked. The patient is usually in no position, since they are ill, to see problems or to notice issues that a family member or close friend would notice. If you notice something, please bring to the attention of the nursing team or the physician.

Stories spread of a caring spouse or friend who averted a consequence to a serious and debilitated patient because of their intervention. I believe this is a very important concept to keep in mind.

Chapter 21

A word on dementia, the most common cause of acute confusion in an elderly adult is urinary tract infection and a change in mental status. When the first thing one must consider is that it's due to urinary tract infection.

However, cardiovascular events, neurological events, and metabolic disorders such as encephalopathy from cirrhosis are not uncommon. Some of the factors that we have been discussing, such as high cholesterol, high blood pressure, or diabetic retinopathy can also impact the brain and be implicated in chronic long-term dementia.

Chapter 22

More reasons to focus on the control of these so that you will not only have a longer life but a better quality. What else can we do in terms of prevention to keep away from hospitals?

1.) Yearly exams including GYN and vision exams

2.) Regular dental exams
3.) Podiatry evaluation if you have a feet problem
4.) Physical therapy if you feel your gait is not steady
5.) Wearing seat belts, helmets, and available, properly fitted protective gear for Sports activities
6.) Fix potential hazards around the house and sidewalks
7.) Put safety guards in the shower if unsteady

The best kind of medicine is preventive medicine and it comes in many forms. Awareness is the key and although it may be a nuisance to implicate some of these strategies, it is often considerably better than being hospitalized with morbidity, mortality, and/or the expense associated with complications.

Aside from the birth of my children and delivering babies, the most rewarding episode in my career again was resuscitating patients outside of the hospital. One of the most dramatic was an elderly overweight man who suffered a heart attack while eating in a restaurant and, for all intents and purposes, was dying. A friend of my wife's, a nurse, and I gave CPI for an extended period of time. While the patient was dying, restaurant patrons formed a circle and prayed. The man was resuscitated. He survived to see many more holidays with his children and grandchildren because of our intervention.

I tell you this story to urge you, if you are able, to spend a day and take a course in CPR. These courses are readily available and can be life-saving. Likewise, if you have access to a defibrillator at work or a public place, don't be afraid to try to use it. It will talk to you and instruct you how to proceed.

At minimum, learn how to take your own pulse, which is found if you trace down from your thumb to your wrist. It should be strong and regular. If your pulse feels irregular, you should proceed to your primary care physician to determine what type of rhythm it is and if it needs to be treated.

Chapter 23

I would also like to discuss topics within the conventional health system and these alternative therapies. Integrative healthcare combines these therapies with alternative therapies. It is an approach that provides many services in a collaborative manner with good communication among healthcare professionals. These services can be delivered at various sites. Some aspects, considered outside of traditional therapy, include nutritional supplements, herbs, massage, chiropractic, yoga, acupuncture, prayer, tai chi, medication, nutrition, and psychosocial therapies.

These therapies are also known as alternative meds, complementary meds, natural meds, or new age meds, although holistic usually refers to more natural remedies, while integrative medicine combines conventional with complementary.

Let's look at some of these therapies.

Chapter 24

As mentioned earlier, herbal medications are medicines made from plants. They have active ingredients, just like conventional medicines. These can harm you if taken improperly. You must also be careful of interactions between herbal medicines and traditional medicines that you may be taking. A challenge with herbals is ensuring there's good quality control and/or they're not contaminated with other products.

Some of the more popular herbs not previously discussed include: Echinacea which is thought to enhance the immune system and is used in the treatment of colds and herpes; Da-huang which is used for constipation; bilberry leaf for diarrhea; Cilantro for insulin resistance; feverfew, which also has both an anti-inflammatory and anti-protozoan effect for fever and/or headaches; ginseng is used for fatigue; ginkgo is thought to have an anti-inflammatory effect, enhance brain health, and is also used for tinnitus; garlic which helps in hypertension and arteriosclerosis; soybeans which lower cholesterol; eucalyptus which is used for cough; basil oil has an antimicrobial effect; and chamomile helps with sleep and anxiety.

Tomato consumption has been touted to lower some levels of cancer and hooked up with other foods and vegetables that are high in the substance cholecopene, and in combination with salt, pimento, and zinc, may support prostate health.

As with supplements, herbal medicine may help patients self-medicate for minor conditions, however, if more serious problems, concerns, or symptoms persist, you should see your family care physician for evaluation of the issue.

Chapter 25

Acupuncture is another tool in an alternative medicine bag. It arises from traditional Chinese medicine in which needles are inserted at certain points. According to traditional Chinese medicine, the body's energy, called Qi, flows through specific channels or meridians.

Whenever Qi is not in balance or blocked, disease may occur. When Qi is blocked, there is an imbalance between the Yin, representing darkness, and Yang, representing light, which are two opposite forces in philosophy; they create a whole whether it be an individual or the universe. There needs to be harmony between these two factors. Each meridian corresponds to an organ group of organs that control bodily functions. When channels are blocked, symptoms occur.

Acupuncture attempts to restore proper flow of energy through the meridians. This is accomplished by placing thin needles into the skin at specific points.

Acupuncture is used in the release of neck pain, back pain, arthritis, and many other medical conditions. And I have seen good results in patients with neuropathies. You can safely use acupuncture with prescription medications. You should make sure that the acupuncturist is licensed and would check with your insurance for coverage issues.

Chapter 26

Chiropractor is a healthcare professional who deals with neuromuscular disorders and emphasizes the body's ability to heal itself. Usually has to do with manipulation but also other forms of alternative therapy.

Massage is the healing of the body's soft tissue. It is helpful in stress management and pain relief. And may help circulation. And many times it is used in combination with aromatherapy. I practice based on the use of essential oils to improve well-being.

Typically aromatherapy is used via inhalation, it is thought to help pain relief, nausea, and stress. Examples are essential oil, tea tree oil, and lavender oil. Prayer and meditation are beneficial in reducing stress, and good alternatives to cues that can lead to destructive behavior. It is thought to lead to an improved consciousness, give insight to the patient, help them become more calm, and lower reactivity to negative events. Prayer can be a very valuable tool in the tool chest. I know there may be critics, but I have experienced how potent it can be for a patient.

Yoga is another spiritual discipline and the practice focuses on bringing harmony to mind and body. It usually works through breathing techniques, posturing, stretch, exercise, meditation. Yoga improves posture, strength, balance, and awareness.

Likewise Tai Chi is a practice of a series of slow general movements, physical posturing, continuous breathing, and meditation. It tries to improve muscle strength, flexibility, and balance.

Less frequently realized is that owning a pet has beneficial health effects, including heart health combats loneliness lowers stress helps social skills.

Chapter 27

Nutrition is an interesting topic in that we live with discussions of nutrition everyday, yet many people find it confusing and overwhelming. . Many patients come to the office for weight reduction and they ask about whether there are newer medications to help suppress appetite. But starving oneself is not necessarily a good idea for the long run. Food is a source of fuel and nutrients for your body.

Basically, carbohydrates come from foods such as grains, starches, vegetables, fruits, milk, bread, and snack foods. They are a source of energy for the body. You need these carbohydrates to increase blood sugar relative to other foods.

Fats are also a type of food that can give you fuel, but fats can be stored. Ingesting too much fat can lead to high cholesterol levels. Fats in the blood are broken down to LDL cholesterol, which is bad, HDL cholesterol, which is good, VLDL, which is bad, and triglycerides, which form a part of a complex called metabolic syndrome. Together, with other risk factors, this leads to diseases. Foods that contain monosaturated or polysaturated fats, which in general are good, or saturated fats or trans fats, which are not so good, for vessel health.

Proteins help the body in building and repairing tissues. With that knowledge in mind, I ask our patients to look at their diet in three ways, since there is not one good fit for all. Each person is an individual with different metabolic needs.

Firstly, what is the food's nutritional value? Is it a good quality product or is it empty calories? Secondly, do you want to be fat or skinny? This is purely calories in and calories out. The third way is more difficult and has to do with the individual's medical issues:

So if you are diabetic, for example, you will want to limit your carbohydrate intakeWhereas, if you have high cholesterol, you might want to limit your fat.

Some relatively healthy diets in general are in the Mediterranean diet. The foundation of this diet is built on vegetables, fruits, herbs, fish, beans, nuts, wheat grain, with only a moderate degree of poultry, eggs, and lean cuts of beef. Another is the DASH diet, utilizing a large amount of vegetable and vegetable oils, fruits, fat-free dairy, fish, poultry, berries, nuts, while limiting fatty meats, sugars, and sodium.

Most people can formulate their own meal plans depending on their age, activity, and comorbidities. Plant proteins are found in dry beans and peas, nuts and soy products. Other sources of protein include meat, fish, poultry, milk, eggs and cheese. Certain diseases are associated with nutritional status.

Anorexia is a condition in which patients take in too little calories for their energy requirements. It is more common in younger females. If unattended, it can lead to serious organ damage.

The opposite end of the spectrum is obesity, which is taking too many calories and storing them as fat. Obesity is related to heart disease, high blood pressure, high cholesterol, diabetes, and sleep apnea.

There may be a relationship for certain cancers. In addition, there are diseases such as Kwashiorkor, Maramus, deficiencies in various nutrients and vitamins that exist. And you may recognize some of the names, pellagra, beriberi, scurvy, and other vitamin deficiencies.

Awareness is the key to a healthy balanced diet, appropriate for your energy expenditure. This will help keep you healthy and help to enhance your immune system.

Chapter 28

Physical therapy is a treatment geared to improve a patient's physical performance. For many elderly patients and patients who have significant medical problems, or post-surgical procedures, there are some disciplines which can be helpful.

Various treatments including range of motion, massage, heat and cold applications, ultrasound, Explanation of biomechanics gait training. The goal is to help relieve pain and strengthen the muscles.

Occupational therapy is a discipline that helps people recover or maintain skills they need to focus to do functions of everyday life. The therapist helps the patient overcome emotional, social, physical problems. The goal is to have the patient become as independent as possible.

Speech therapy can help people with difficulty speaking by increasing pronunciation, strengthening muscles of speech. Skilled nursing can help with medications. evaluation, wound care, education, and communication with the health system on behalf of the patient.

Chapter 29

I've talked about my personal evolution, the evolution of the health system, and now I'd like to make a comment about, I believe, where the evolution of science and medicine is going.

Since the cell was discovered in 1665 with a microscope, and then the nucleus of the cell, was discovered, which contains all of our chromosomes, the biochemists have been able to examine it, and found it to be the repository of DNA. DNA is a complex molecule, that is, DNA contains all information to build and maintain an organism. All living things have DNA with few exceptions within their cells. DNA makes genes and genes make chromosomes.

Some genes make proteins for body functions. Others regulate other parts of the genetic system, turning other genes on or off for specific purposes. Some produce substances that perform specific tasks in the body.

Most genes are the same. in All people, but there's a small amount.that is different and unique and this is what gives us our different physical features. The Human Genome Project is working to sequence all of human DNA. Once you've had these sequences, and with the help of supercomputers and AI, you can see the logical conclusion of what the future will be, which is able to manipulate the genes, turn some on, turn some off, or affect the substances that they make. We've already seen the beginning of this process in targeted studies therapies and stem cell therapy, for example, and various disorders.

This is where I believe medicine is headed, and there will be a dramatic change in how medicine will be individualized and delivered.

Much of the information in this book comes mostly from personal experience, but some comes from recommendations from organizations , agencies, various reference sources and double-blinded studies, which are studies in clinical trials in which neither the researcher nor the patients know what treatment. or intervention is being given until the trial is over.

In the old system that I have described, family, staff, friends, and myself formed a lasting bond among ourselves which continues to this day with our goal to give the best possible medical care for our patients. Everyone worked hard and supported each other, and although the days were long, the environment was mostly happy.

Contrast this to the present system, where there is a significant amount of stress and mediocrity present, many physicians are disenchanted. Due to the loss of autonomy, emphasis on computerization and reimbursement rather than medical care, staff are often overwhelmed by all the demands placed on them by insurers and agencies.

Unfortunately, my vision of future visits is even more disturbing. With the evolution of artificial intelligence and supercomputing, I worry about the patient-doctor relationship being overrun by "big brother, " who listens in on the conversation and gives treatment based on hard facts with no consideration for the spiritual or emotional needs of the patient. We should be wary of a medical system that leaves no place for empathy, sympathy, and no intrapersonal trust-building relationship between doctor and patient.

Chapter 30

Chapter [Insert #]

Additional Potential Topics/Chapters/Vlogs:

1. How can patients ensure a doctor isn't just selling them procedures?

   [Insert Answers]

2. How can I recognize a solidly credentialed, knowledgeable, experienced doctor for a new exam?

   [Insert Answers]

3. How do you think the decline in private practice will impact patient outcomes over time?

   [Insert Answers]

4. How do you ensure you are practicing in a way that remains unbiased toward women and minorities?

   [Insert Answers]

5. How do we provide the growing number of doctors needed to treat the aged?

   [Insert Answers]

6. How do you feel about conservative or alternative therapies to medicine?

   [Insert Answers]

7. What does integrative medicine mean to you?

   [Insert Answers]

www.ingramcontent.com/pod-product-compliance
Lightning Source LLC
LaVergne TN
LVHW070956210926
848482LV00002B/225

8. **What kind of Healthcare system would doctors themselves like to see?**

[Insert Answers]